Easy Keto Vegetarian Recipes

Fast and Easy Vegetarian Ketogenic Recipes to Lose Weight on a Budget

Lidia Wong

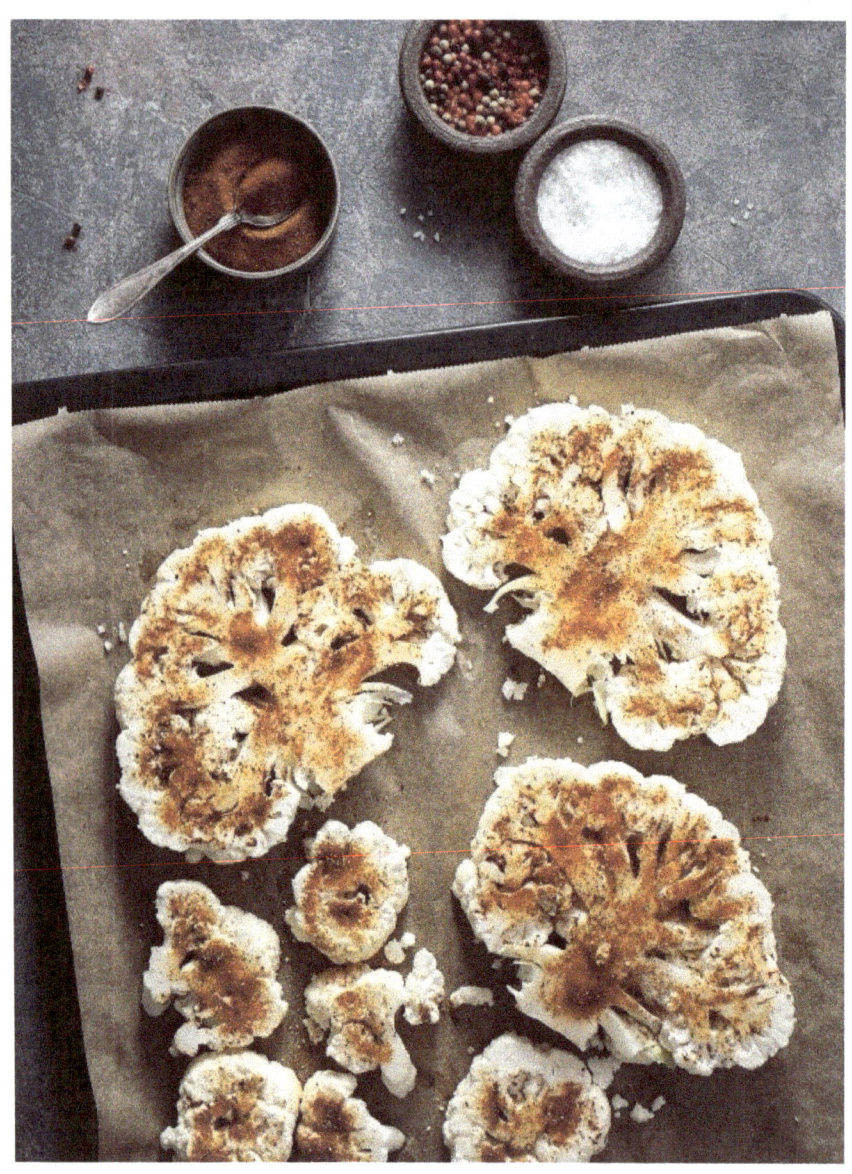

© **Copyright 2021 by Lidia Wong - All rights reserved.**

The content contained within this book may not be reproduced, duplicated or transmitted without direct written permission from the author or the publisher.
Under no circumstances will any blame or legal responsibility be held against the publisher, or author, for any damages, reparation, or monetary loss due to the information contained within this book. Either directly or indirectly.

Legal Notice:
This book is copyright protected. This book is only for personal use. You cannot amend, distribute, sell, use, quote or paraphrase any part, or the content within this book, without the consent of the author or publisher.

Disclaimer Notice:
Please note the information contained within this document is for educational and entertainment purposes only. All effort has been executed to present accurate, up to date, and reliable, complete information. No warranties of any kind are declared or implied. Readers acknowledge that the author is not engaging in the rendering of legal, financial, medical or professional advice. The content within this book has been derived from various sources. Please consult a licensed professional before attempting any techniques outlined in this book.
By reading this document, the reader agrees that under no circumstances is the author responsible for any losses, direct or indirect, which are incurred as a result of the use of information contained within this document, including, but not limited to, — errors, omissions, or inaccuracies.

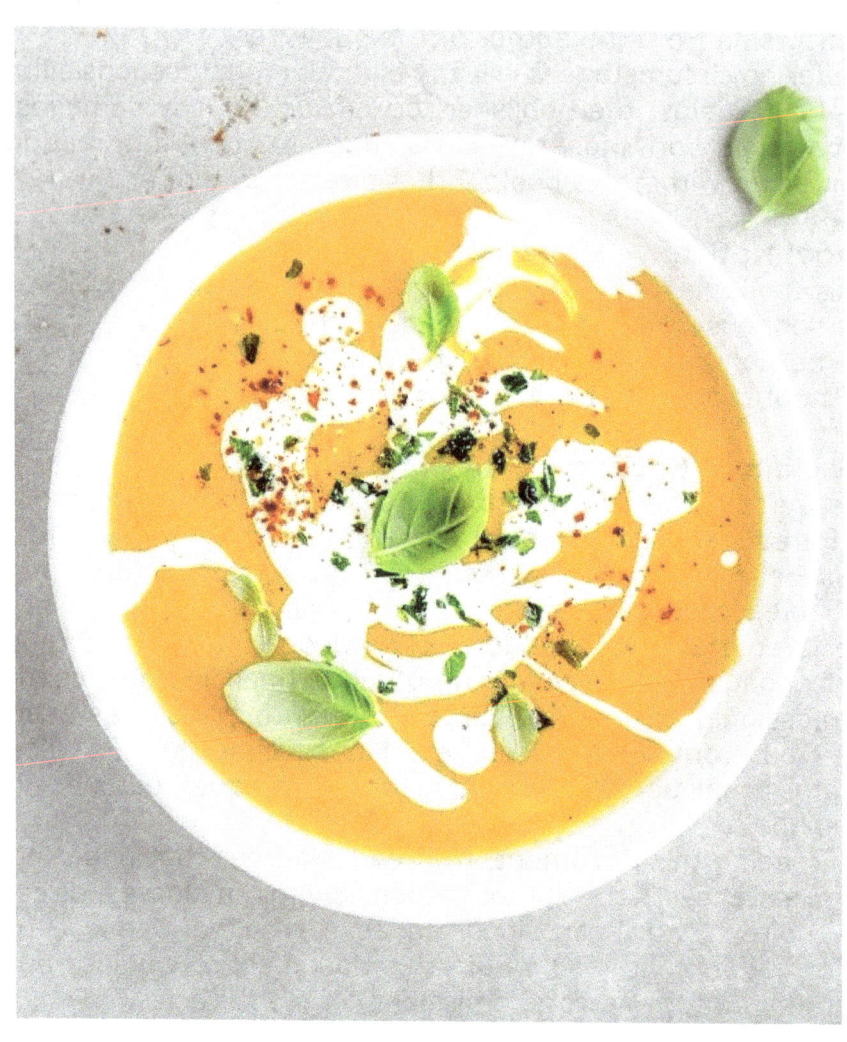

TABLE OF CONTENTS

INTRODUCTION 1

Waffle/Cinnamon Roll 3

Keto Flax Cinnamon Muffins 6

Eggfast Muffins (ovo) 8

Mushroom and Mustard Greens Mix 10

Chard and Garlic Sauce 12

Kale and Raisins 14

Veggie Hash 15

Creamy Cauliflower Spinach Soup 17

Creamy Squash Soup 19

Low-Carb Jambalaya 21

Vegan Potstickers 23

Tofu Loco Moco 25

Pimiento Tofu balls 28

Peppers and Celery Sauté 30

Cauliflower Salad 32

Baked Broccoli and Pine Nuts 33

Glazed Cauliflower 35

Sweet Potatoes Side Dish 36

- Rustic Mashed Potatoes ... 38
- Glazed Carrots ... 40
- Eggplant And Kale Mix ... 42
- Turmeric Coconut Rice Mix ... 44
- Baked Eggplant ... 45
- Avocado Salad ... 47
- Creamy Celery Soup ... 49
- Curried Butternut And Red Lentil Soup With Chard ... 51
- Spinach, Walnut, And Apple Soup ... 53
- Tuscan White Bean Soup ... 55
- Cream of Tomato Soup ... 58
- Chickpea, Tomato, And Eggplant Stew ... 60
- Creamy Garlic Mushrooms with Angel Hair Shirataki ... 62
- Tofu and Spinach Lasagna with Red Sauce ... 65
- Creamy Mushrooms with Shirataki ... 69
- Corn And Red Bean Salad ... 71
- Stuffed Avocado ... 73
- Spinach and Pomegranate Salad ... 75
- Avocado And Tempeh Bacon Wraps ... 76
- Veggie Spread ... 78
- Tomato and Watermelon Bites ... 80

Keto Almond Zucchini Bread 81
Fathead Crackers 83
Asian Cucumber Salad 85
Tangerine Stew 86
Warm Rum Butter Spiced Cider 87
Mango Rice Pudding. 88
Tapioca With Apricots. 90
Candied Pecans 91
Vanilla Pudding 93
Lime Cherries and Rice Pudding 95
Green Tea Coconut Cake 97
Cherries Stew 99
Raspberry Chia Pudding 100

NOTE **101**

INTRODUCTION

The keto diet is the shortened term for ketogenic diet and it is essentially a high-fat and low-carb diet that helps you lose weight, thereby bringing various health benefits. This diet drastically restricts your carb intake while increasing your fat intake; this pushes your body to go into a state know as "*ketosis*". We will tackle ketosis in a bit.

The human body uses glucose from carbs to fuel metabolic pathways—meaning various bodily functions like digestion, breathing, etc.. Essentially, anything that needs energy. Even when you are resting, the body needs fuel or energy for you to continue living. If you think about it, when have you ever stopped breathing, or your heart stopped beating, or your liver stopped from cleansing the body, or your kidneys from filtering blood?

Never, unless you're dead, which is the only time in which the body doesn't need energy. In normal circumstances, glucose is the primary pathway when it comes to sourcing the body's energy.

But the body also has another pathway; it can utilize fats to fuel the various bodily processes. And this is what we call "*ketosis*". And the body can only enter ketosis when there is no glucose available, thus the reason for sticking to a low-carb diet is essential in the keto diet. Since no glucose is available, the body is pushed to use fats—it can either come from the food you consume or from your body's fat reserves—the adipose tissue or from the flabby parts of your body. This is how the keto diet helps you lose weight, by burning up all those stored fats that you have and using it to fuel bodily processes.

That said, if for whatever reason you are a vegetarian, following a ketogenic diet can be extremely difficult. A vegetarian diet is largely free of animal products, which means that food tends to be usually high in carbohydrates. Still, with careful planning, it is possible. This Cookbook will provide you with various easy and delicious dishes to help you stick to your ketogenic diet plan while being a vegetarian.

Enjoy!

Waffle/Cinnamon Roll

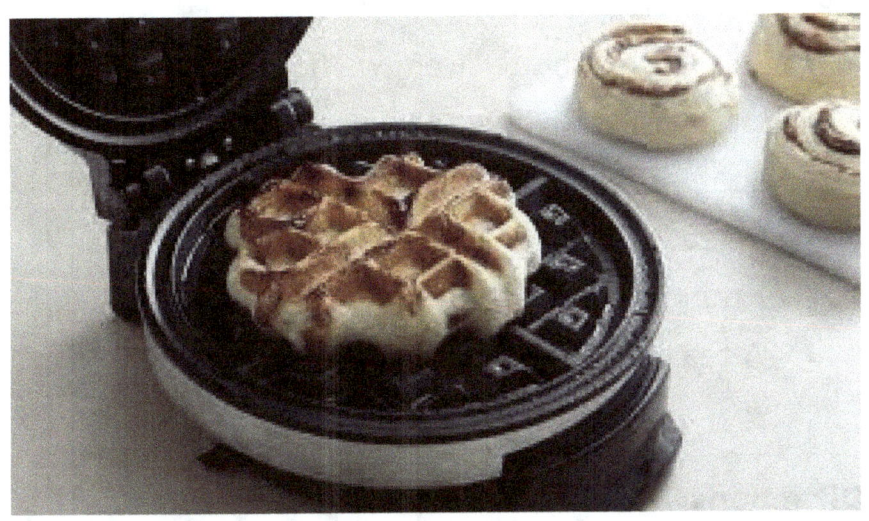

Preparation Time: 5 minutes

Cooking Time: 6 minutes

Servings: 1

Ingredients:

Waffle:

- ½ teaspoon vanilla extract
- 2 large eggs
- ½ teaspoon cinnamon
- ¼ teaspoon baking soda

- 1 tablespoon erythritol
- 6 tablespoons almond flour

Frosting:

- 2 teaspoons batter from waffles
- 1 tablespoon heavy cream
- 2 tablespoons cream cheese
- ¼ teaspoon of cinnamon
- 1 tablespoon erythritol
- ¼ teaspoon vanilla extract

Directions:

1. Add all the dry waffle ingredients in a mixing bowl. In another mixing bowl, mix your wet ingredients.
2. Ensure that they are combined well.
3. Add your wet ingredients to the dry ingredients and blend well.
4. Heat your waffle iron. When the waffle iron is hot, add your batter.
5. Remember to reserve 2 teaspoons of your waffle batter for the frosting.
6. While the waffle is cooking, add your cream cheese and erythritol to a small bowl.
7. Now add heavy cream, cinnamon, and batter.

8. Mix until smooth.
9. Once the waffle is finished cooking, remove it from iron, place on serving the dish and spread frosting on top.
10. Enjoy!

Nutritional Values (Per Serving):

Calories: 545 Fat: 52 g Carbs: 6 g Protein: 25 g

Keto Flax Cinnamon Muffins

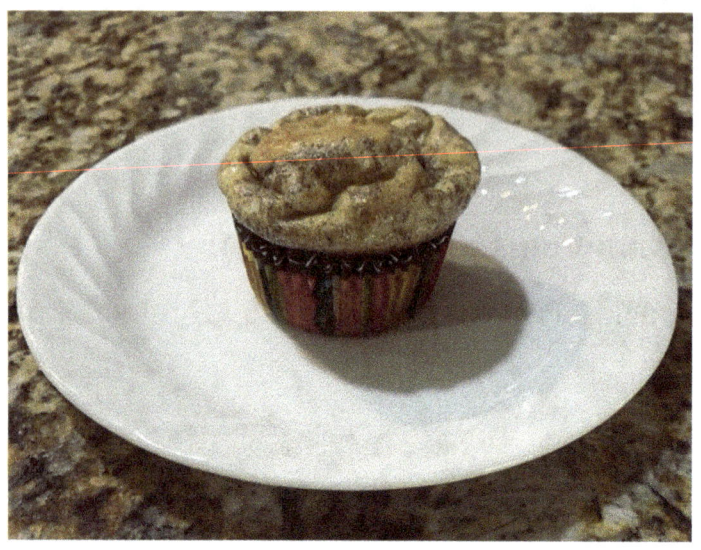

Preparation Time: 10 minutes

Cooking Time: 20 minutes

Servings: 12

Ingredients:

- 4 organic eggs, beaten
- 1 cup flax seed, ground
- ½ cup olive oil
- ½ cup coconut sugar
- ¼ cup coconut flour

- 1/8 teaspoon salt
- 2 teaspoons vanilla
- 2 teaspoons cinnamon
- 1 teaspoon lemon juice
- ½ teaspoon baking soda
- 1 cup walnuts, chopped

Directions:
1. Preheat your oven to 350°Fahrenheit.
2. Spray muffin pan with cooking spray and set aside.
3. Add all ingredients into a mixing bowl and mix well to combine.
4. Pour the batter into prepared muffin pan—filling each about ¾ full of mixture.
5. Bake for about 20 minutes.
6. Serve and enjoy!

Nutritional Values (Per Serving):

Calories: 219 Fat: 20 g Carbohydrates: 6 g Sugar: 1 g Protein: 6 g Cholesterol: 55 mg

Eggfast Muffins (ovo)

Preparation Time: 15 minutes

Cooking Time: 25 minutes

Servings: 9

Ingredients:

- 9 large organic eggs
- ¼ cup fresh parsley (chopped)
- 1 cup mushrooms (sliced)
- ½ cup scallions (finely chopped)
- 1 cup broccoli florets (stems removed)
- 4 tbsp. sugar-free sweet hot sauce
- Sea salt and pepper to taste

Directions:

1. Preheat oven to 375°F / 190°C, and line a 9-cup muffin tray with muffin liners.
2. Take a large bowl, crack the eggs in it, and whisk while adding salt and pepper to taste.
3. Add all the remaining ingredients to the bowl and stir thoroughly.
4. Fill each muffin liner with the egg mixture.

Repeat this for all 9 muffins.
5. Transfer the tray to the oven and bake for about 30 minutes, or until the muffins have risen and browned on top.
6. Take the tray out of the oven, and let the muffins cool down for about 2 minutes; serve and enjoy.
7. Alternatively, store the muffins in an airtight container in the fridge, and consume within 3 days.
8. Store for a maximum of 30 days in the freezer and thaw at room temperature. Use a microwave, toaster oven, or pan to reheat the omelet.

Nutrition:

Calories: 76kcal, Net Carbs: 1.1g, Fat: 4.9g, Protein: 6.9g. Fiber: 0.4g, Sugar: 0.6g

Mushroom and Mustard Greens Mix

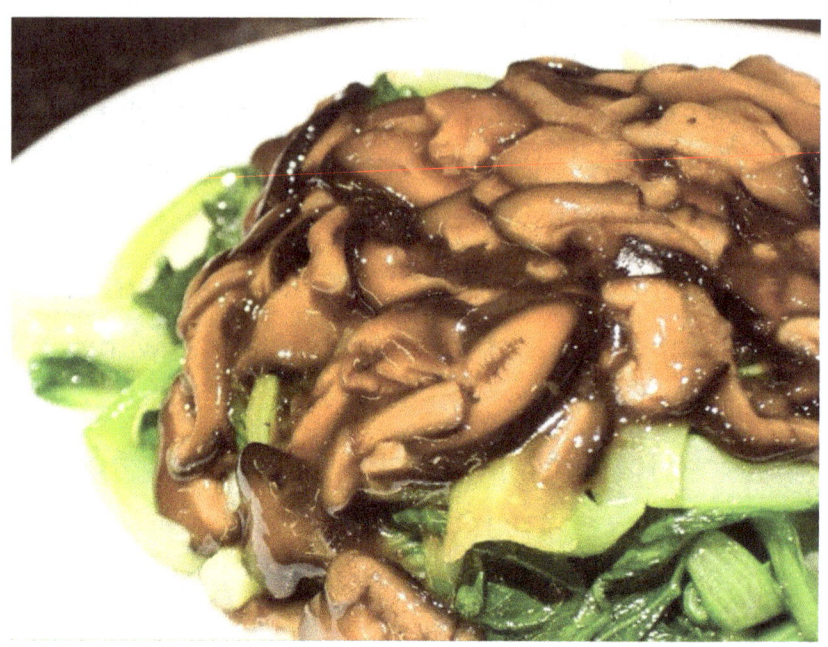

Preparation time: 10 minutes

Cooking time: 20 minutes

Servings: 4

Ingredients:

- 2 cups mustard greens
- 1 pound white mushrooms, halved
- 1 tablespoon lime juice

- 3 scallions, chopped
- 2 tablespoons olive oil
- 1 teaspoon rosemary, dried
- 1 teaspoon sweet paprika
- 2 bunches parsley, chopped
- 3 garlic cloves, minced
- Salt and black pepper to the taste

Directions:

1. Heat up a pan with the oil over medium heat, add the scallions, paprika, garlic and parsley and sauté for 5 minutes.
2. Add the mushrooms and the other ingredients, toss, cook over medium heat for 15 minutes, divide between plates and serve.

Nutrition:

calories 76, fat 1, fiber 2, carbs 3, protein 3

Chard and Garlic Sauce

Preparation time: 10 minutes

Cooking time: 15 minutes

Servings: 4

Ingredients:

- ½ cup walnuts, chopped
- 4 cups red chard, torn
- 3 tablespoons olive oil
- 1 celery stalks, chopped
- 1 cup coconut cream
- 4 garlic cloves, minced
- Juice of 1 lime
- 1 tablespoon balsamic vinegar
- 2/3 cup scallions, chopped
- A pinch of sea salt and black pepper

Directions:

1. Heat up a pan with the oil over medium heat, add the scallions, garlic and the celery and sauté for 5 minutes.

2. Add the chard and the other ingredients, toss, cook over medium heat for 10 minutes more, divide between plates and serve.

Nutrition:

calories 374, fat 34.2, fiber 6.7, carbs 15.4, protein 9

Kale and Raisins

Preparation time: 10 minutes

Cooking time: 20 minutes

Servings: 4

Ingredients:

- 1 pound kale, torn
- 1 tomato, cubed
- ¼ cup raisins
- 2 tablespoons avocado oil
- Juice of 1 lime
- 1 teaspoon nutmeg, ground
- ½ teaspoon ginger, grated
- ½ teaspoon cinnamon powder
- 1 tablespoon chives, chopped
- A pinch of sea salt and black pepper

Directions:

1. Heat up a pan with the oil over medium heat, add the kale, tomato, lime juice and the other ingredients, toss, cook for 20 minutes, divide into bowls and serve.

Nutrition:

calories 102, fat 1.2, fiber 2.7, carbs 21.4, protein 4

Veggie Hash

Preparation time: 10 minutes

Cooking time: 20 minutes

Servings: 4

Ingredients:

- 1 bunch asparagus, chopped
- 1 shallot, chopped
- 2 cups radishes, halved
- ½ cup mushrooms, halved
- 3 tablespoons olive oil
- ½ cup roasted bell peppers, chopped
- 2 garlic cloves, minced
- A pinch of salt and black pepper
- 1 tablespoon chives, chopped
- 1 tablespoon sage, chopped

Directions:

1. Heat up a pan with the oil over medium heat, add the shallot and the garlic and sauté for 5 minutes.

2. Add the mushrooms and sauté for 5 minutes more.
3. Add the rest of the ingredients, toss, cook everything over medium heat for another 10 minutes, divide into bowls and serve.

Nutrition:

calories 135, fat 2, fiber 4, carbs 5.4, protein 5

Creamy Cauliflower Spinach Soup

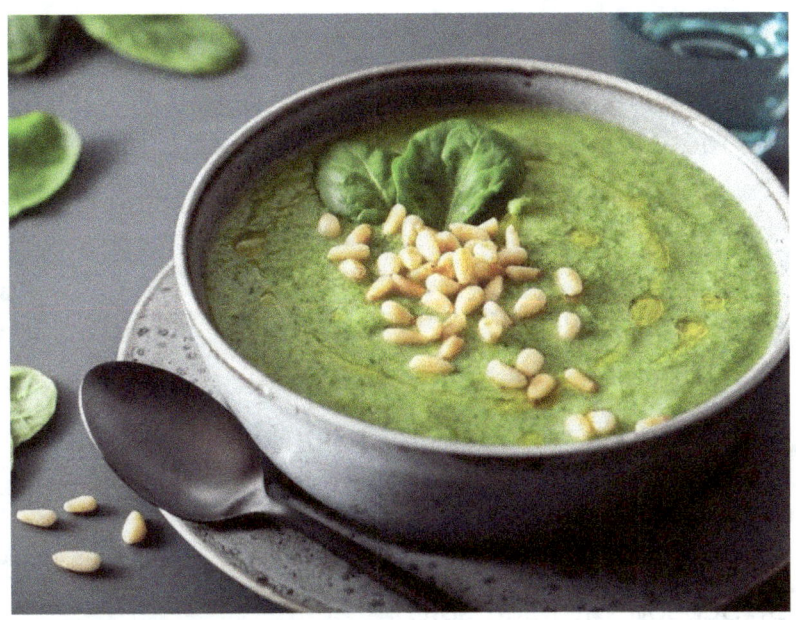

Preparation Time: 10 minutes

Cooking Time: 35 minutes

Servings: 5

Ingredients:

- 5 watercress, chopped
- 1 lb. cauliflower, chopped
- 8 cups vegetable broth
- 5-ounces spinach, fresh, chopped

- ½ cup coconut milk
- Sea salt

Directions:

1. Add cauliflower along with broth to a large pot over medium heat for 15 minutes, bring to a boil.
2. Add spinach and watercress, cook for another 10 minutes.
3. Remove from heat and using a blender puree the soup until smooth.
4. Add coconut milk and stir well.
5. Season with sea salt.
6. Serve hot and enjoy!

Nutritional Values (Per Serving):

Calories: 153 Cholesterol: 0 mg Sugar: 4.3 g Fat: 8.3 g Carbohydrates: 8.7 g Protein: 11.9 g

Creamy Squash Soup

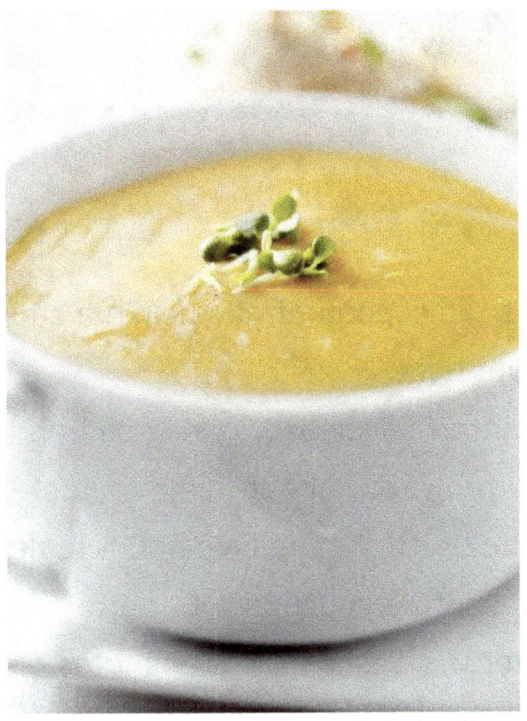

Preparation Time: 10 minutes

Cooking Time: 35 minutes

Servings: 8

Ingredients:

- 1 lb. butternut squash, peeled, diced
- 5 tablespoons extra-virgin olive oil

- 4 cups vegetable broth
- 3 garlic cloves, minced
- 2 bay leaves
- ½ cup heavy cream
- 1 teaspoon salt

Directions:

1. Heat 1 tablespoon of olive oil in a saucepan over medium heat.
2. Add butternut squash, garlic, salt and sauté until lightly browned. About five minutes.
3. Add the broth, bay leaves and 4 tablespoons of olive oil into a saucepan. Bring to a boil.
4. Simmer the squash for 30 minutes or until it is completely cooked.
5. Discard the bay leaves. Using blender puree the soup until smooth.
6. Add heavy cream and stir well.
7. Serve warm and enjoy!

Nutritional Values (Per Serving):

Calories: 147 Fat: 12.3 g Cholesterol: 10 mg Sugar: 1.6 g Carbohydrates: 7.7 g Protein: 3.2 g

Low-Carb Jambalaya

Preparation Time: 10 min

Cooking Time: 10 min

Serves: 4

Ingredients:

- 200 grams Seitan Sausages, chopped
- 400 grams Cauliflower, riced
- 1 Red Bell Pepper, diced
- 1 cup Vegetable Broth
- ¼ cup Frozen Peas
- 3 cloves Garlic, minced
- ½ White Onion, diced
- 3 tbsp Olive Oil
- 1 tsp Paprika
- 1 tsp Oregano
- Salt and Pepper, to taste

Directions:

1. Heat olive oil in a pot.
2. Add seitan and sear until slightly brown.

3. Add garlic, onions, and bell pepper. Sautee until aromatic.
4. Add cauliflower, broth, oregano, paprika, salt, and pepper.
5. Simmer for 5 minutes
6. Serve hot.

Nutritional Values:

Kcal per serve: 200 Fat: 15 g. Protein: 10 g. Carbs: 9 g.

Vegan Potstickers

Preparation Time: 25 min

Cooking Time: 5 min

Serves: 8

Ingredients:

- 250 grams Firm Tofu, pressed and crumbled
- ½ cup Diced Shiitake Mushrooms
- ¼ cup Finely Chopped Carrots
- ¼ cup Finely Chopped Spring Onions
- 2 tbsp Soy Sauce
- 1 tsp Minced Ginger
- 1 tbsp Sesame Oil
- 2 tbsp Peanut Oil, plus more for pan-frying
- 1/2 tsp Salt
- ½ tsp Pepper
- 250 grams Green Cabbage

Directions:

1. Heat peanut oil in a pan. Sautee minced ginger and spring onions until aromatic.

2. Add tofu, mushrooms, and carrots. Sautee for 2-3 minutes.
3. Take off the heat and season with soy sauce, sesame oil, salt, and pepper.
4. Blanch cabbage leaves in boiling water to soften.
5. Lay a piece cabbage leaf on your chopping board. Fill with about a tablespoon of the tofu mixture. Fold and secure with toothpicks.
6. Repeat for remaining ingredients.
7. Heat about 2 tbsp of peanut oil in a pan. Arrange dumplings in and fry for 2 minutes over medium heat.
8. Add about a quarter cup of water into the pan and cover. Steam over low heat until all water has evaporated.

Nutritional Values:

Kcal per serve: 118 Fat: 9 g. Protein: 9 g. Carbs: 5 g.

Tofu Loco Moco

Preparation Time: 12 minutes

Cooking Time: 28 minutes

Serving: 4

Ingredients:

For the loco moco patties:

- 1 ½ lb tofu, crumbled
- 1/3 cup almond meal
- ½ tsp nutmeg powder
- 1 tsp onion powder
- 1 large egg
- 2 tbsp cashew cream
- Salt and black pepper to taste
- 3 tbsp avocado oil

For the mushroom gravy:

- 1 tbsp salted butter
- 1 shallot, finely chopped
- 1 cup sliced oyster mushrooms
- 2 tsp tamarind sauce
- 1 cup vegetable stock
- Salt and black pepper to taste

- ½ tsp arrowroot starch

For the fried eggs:

- 2 tbsp olive oil
- 4 large eggs
- Salt and black pepper to taste

Directions:

For the loco moco patties:

1. In a large bowl, combine the tofu, almond meal, nutmeg powder, onion powder, salt, and black pepper. In a small bowl, whisk the eggs with the cashew cream and mix into the tofu mixture until the batter is sticky. Form 8 patties from the mixture.
2. Heat the avocado oil in a medium skillet over medium heat and fry the patties in batches on both sides until compacted and cooked through, 16 minutes. Transfer to a serving plate and set aside.

For the mushroom gravy:

3. Melt the butter in the same skillet and cook the shallot and mushrooms until softened, 7 minutes.

4. Meanwhile, in a medium bowl, combine the remaining ingredients and pour the mixture into the skillet. Cook until slightly thickened, 3 minutes.
5. Turn the heat off and set aside.

For the fried eggs:

6. Heat half of the olive oil in a small skillet, crack in an egg, and fry sunshine style, 1 minute. Plate and fry the remaining eggs in the same manner. Season with salt and black pepper.
7. Serve the tofu with the mushroom gravy and the fried rice.

Nutrition:

Calories: 258, Total Fat: 21g, Saturated Fat: 13.5g, Total Carbs: 16 g, Dietary Fiber: 6g, Sugar: 7g, Protein: 6g, Sodium: 37 mg

Pimiento Tofu balls

Preparation Time: 10 minutes

Cooking Time: 15 minutes

Serving: 4

Ingredients:

- ¼ cup chopped pimientos
- 1/3 cup mayonnaise
- 3 tbsp cashew cream
- 1 tsp paprika powder
- 1 tbsp Dijon mustard
- 1 pinch cayenne pepper
- 4 oz grated Parmesan cheese
- 1 ½ lbs. tofu, pressed and crumbled
- Salt and black pepper to taste
- 1 large egg
- 2 tbsp olive oil, for frying

Directions:

1. In a large bowl, add all the Ingredients except for the olive oil and with gloves on your hands, mix the Ingredients until well combined.

2. Form bite size balls from the mixture.
3. Heat the olive oil in a medium non-stick skillet and fry the tofu balls in batches on both sides until brown and cooked through, 4 to 5 minutes on each side.
4. Transfer the tofu balls to a serving plate and serve warm.

Nutrition:

Calories:254, Total Fat: 36.8g, Saturated Fat: 8.7g, Total Carbs: 12g, Dietary Fiber: 1g, Sugar: 1g, Protein:26 g, Sodium:773 mg

Peppers and Celery Sauté

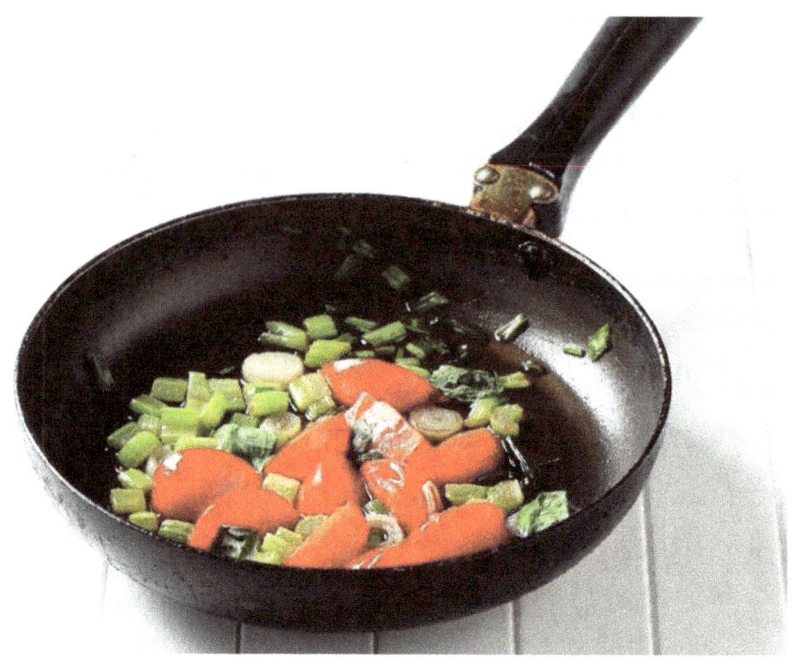

Preparation time: 10 minutes

Cooking time: 15 minutes

Servings: 4

Ingredients:

- 1 green bell pepper, cut into medium chunks
- 1 red bell pepper, cut into medium chunks

- 1 celery stalk, chopped
- 2 scallions, chopped
- 2 tablespoons olive oil
- 1 tablespoons parsley, chopped
- 1 teaspoon cumin, ground
- Salt and black pepper to the taste
- 2 garlic cloves, minced

Directions:

1. Heat up a pan with the oil over medium heat, add the scallions, garlic and cumin and sauté for 5 minutes.
2. Add the peppers, celery and the other ingredients, toss, cook over medium heat for 10 minutes more, divide between plates and serve.

Nutrition:

calories 87, fat 2.4, fiber 3, carbs 5, protein 4

Cauliflower Salad

Preparation time: 10 minutes

Cooking time: 0 minutes

Servings: 4

Ingredients:

- 1 pound cauliflower florets, blanched
- 1 avocado, peeled, pitted and cubed
- 1 cup spring onions, chopped
- 1 tablespoon lime juice
- 1 tablespoon chives, chopped
- 1 cup kalamata olives, pitted and halved
- Salt and black pepper to the taste

Directions:

1. In a bowl, combine the cauliflower florets with the avocado and the other ingredients, toss and serve as a side salad.

Nutrition:

calories 211, fat 20, fiber 2, carbs 3, protein 4

Baked Broccoli and Pine Nuts

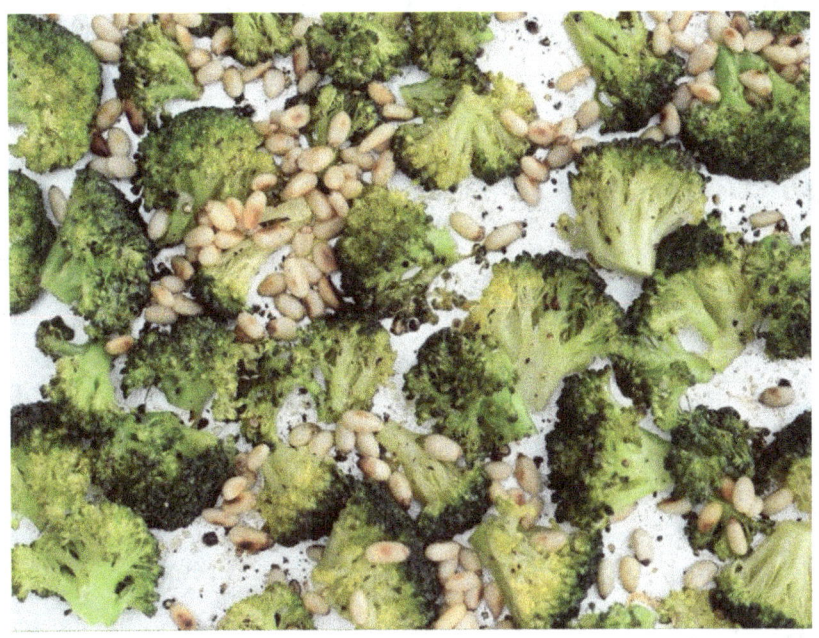

Preparation time: 10 minutes

Cooking time: 30 minutes

Servings: 4

Ingredients:

- 1 pound broccoli florets
- 2 tablespoons olive oil
- 1 tablespoon garlic, minced

- 1 tablespoon pine nuts, toasted
- 1 tablespoon lemon juice
- 2 teaspoons mustard
- A pinch of salt and black pepper

Directions:

1. In a roasting pan, combine the broccoli with the oil, the garlic and the other ingredients, toss and bake at 380 degrees F for 30 minutes.
2. Divide everything between plates and serve as a side dish.

Nutrition:

calories 220, fat 6, fiber 2, carbs 7, protein 6

Glazed Cauliflower

Preparation time: 10 minutes

Cooking time: 25 minutes

Servings: 4

Ingredients:

- 1 tablespoon olive oil
- 1 teaspoon chili powder
- 1 pound cauliflower florets
- 1 tablespoon maple syrup
- 1 tablespoon rosemary, chopped
- A pinch of salt and black pepper

Directions:

1. Spread the cauliflower on a baking sheet lined with parchment paper, add the oil and the other ingredients, toss and cook in the oven at 375 degrees F for 25 minutes.
2. Divide the mix between plates and serve.

Nutrition:

calories 76, fat 3.9, fiber 3.4, carbs 10.3, protein 2.4

Sweet Potatoes Side Dish

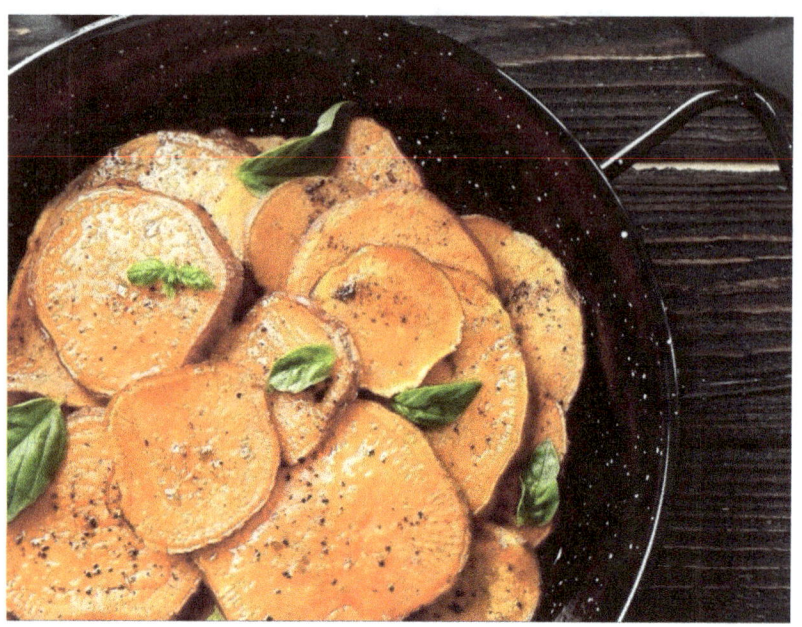

Preparation time: 10 minutes

Cooking time: 3 hours

Servings: 10

Ingredients:

- 4 pounds sweet potatoes, thinly sliced
- ½ cup orange juice
- 3 tablespoons stevia

- A pinch of salt and black pepper
- ½ teaspoon thyme, dried
- ½ teaspoon sage, dried
- 2 tablespoons olive oil

Directions:

1. Arrange potato slices on the bottom of your slow cooker.
2. In a bowl, mix orange juice with salt, pepper, stevia, thyme, sage and oil and whisk well.
3. Add this over potatoes, cover slow cooker and cook on High for 3 hours.
4. Divide between plates and serve as a side dish.
5. Enjoy!

Nutrition:

calories 189, fat 4, fiber 4, carbs 36, protein 4

Rustic Mashed Potatoes

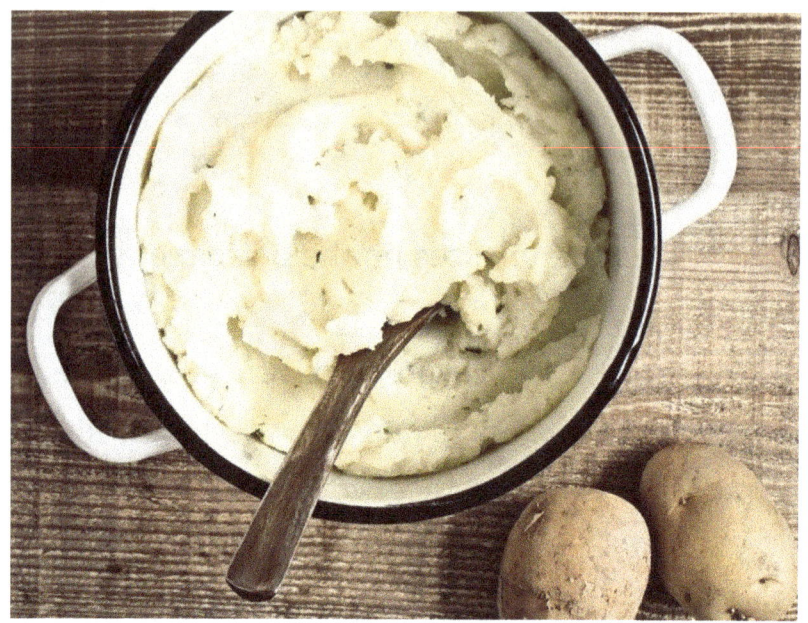

Preparation time: 10 minutes

Cooking time: 4 hours

Servings: 6

Ingredients:

- 1 bay leaf
- 6 garlic cloves, peeled
- 3 pounds gold potatoes, peeled and cubed
- 1 cup coconut milk

- 28 ounces veggie stock
- 3 tablespoons olive oil
- Salt and black pepper to the taste

Directions:

1. In your slow cooker, mix potatoes with stock, bay leaf, garlic, salt and pepper, cover and cook on High for 4 hours.
2. Drain potatoes and garlic, return them to your slow cooker and mash using a potato masher.
3. Add oil and coconut milk, whisk well, divide between plates and serve as a side dish.
4. Enjoy!

Nutrition:

calories 135, fat 5, fiber 1, carbs 20, protein 3

Glazed Carrots

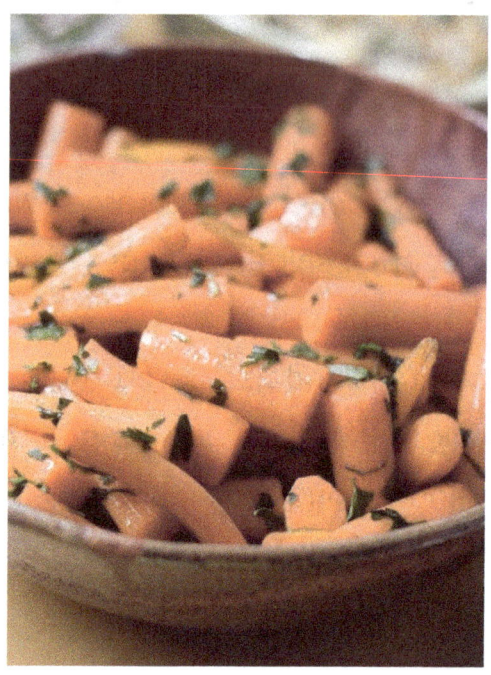

Preparation time: 10 minutes

Cooking time: 4 hours

Servings: 10

Ingredients:

- 2 tablespoons orange peel, shredded
- 1 pound parsnips, cut into medium chunks
- 2 pounds carrots, cut into medium chunks

- 1 cup orange juice
- ½ cup orange marmalade
- ½ cup veggie stock
- 1 tablespoon tapioca, crushed
- A pinch of salt and black pepper
- 3 tablespoons olive oil
- ¼ cup parsley, chopped

Directions:

1. In your slow cooker, mix parsnips with carrots.
2. In a bowl, mix orange peel with orange juice, stock, orange marmalade, tapioca, salt and pepper, whisk and add over carrots.
3. Cover slow cooker and cook everything on High for 4 hours.
4. Add parsley, toss, divide between plates and serve as a side dish.
5. Enjoy!

Nutrition:

calories 159, fat 4, fiber 4, carbs 30, protein 2

Eggplant And Kale Mix

Preparation time: 10 minutes

Cooking time: 2 hours

Servings: 6

Ingredients:

- 14 ounces canned roasted tomatoes and garlic
- 4 cups eggplant, cubed
- 1 yellow bell pepper, chopped
- 1 red onion, cut into medium wedges
- 4 cups kale leaves
- 2 tablespoons olive oil
- 1 teaspoon mustard
- 3 tablespoons red vinegar
- 1 garlic clove, minced
- A pinch of salt and black pepper
- ½ cup basil, chopped

Directions:

1. In your slow cooker, mix eggplant cubes with canned tomatoes, bell pepper and onion, toss, cover and cook on High for 2 hours.

2. Add kale, toss, cover slow cooker and leave aside for now.
3. Meanwhile, in a bowl, mix oil with vinegar, mustard, garlic, salt and pepper and whisk well.
4. Add this over eggplant mix, also add basil, toss, divide between plates and serve as a side dish.
5. Enjoy!

Nutrition:

calories 251, fat 9, fiber 6, carbs 34, protein 8

Turmeric Coconut Rice Mix

Preparation time: 10 minutes

Cooking time: 20 minutes

Servings: 4

Ingredients:

- 1 cup cauliflower rice
- 1 tablespoon coconut cream
- 1 cup coconut milk
- 1 teaspoon turmeric powder
- ½ teaspoon garam masala
- A pinch of salt and black pepper
- 1 tablespoon cilantro, chopped

Directions:

1. Put the coconut milk in a pan, heat up over medium heat, add the rice, cream and the other ingredients, toss, cook for 20 minutes, divide between plates and serve.

Nutrition:

calories 211, fat 5, fiber 4, carbs 6, protein 12

Baked Eggplant

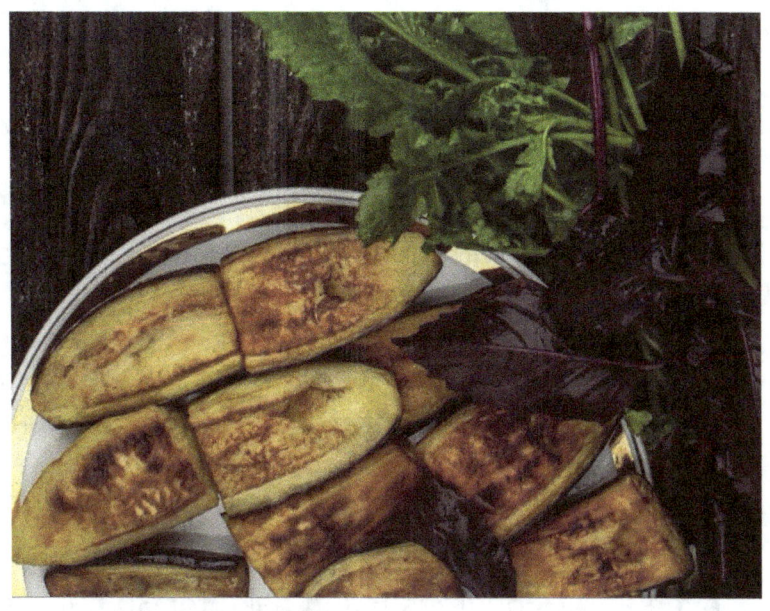

Preparation time: 10 minutes

Cooking time: 30 minutes

Servings: 3

Ingredients:

- 2 eggplants, sliced
- A pinch of sea salt
- Black pepper to taste
- 1 cup almonds, ground

- 1 teaspoon garlic, minced
- 2 teaspoons olive oil

Directions:

1. Grease a baking dish with some of the oil and arrange eggplant slices on it.
2. Season them with a pinch of salt and some black pepper and leave them aside for 10 minutes.
3. In a food processor, mix almonds with the rest of the oil, garlic, a pinch of salt and black pepper and blend well.
4. Spread this over eggplant slices, place in the oven at 425 degrees F and bake for 30 minutes.
5. Divide between plates and serve.
6. Enjoy!

Nutritional value/serving:

calories 303, fat 19,6, fiber 16,9, carbs 28,6, protein 10,3

Avocado Salad

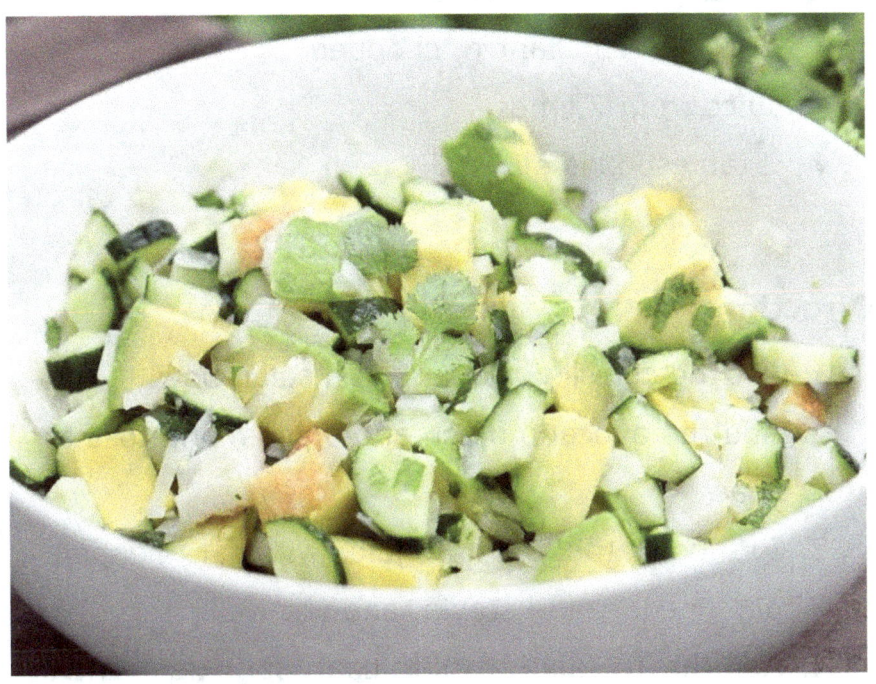

Preparation time: 10 minutes

Cooking time: 0 minutes

Servings: 4

Ingredients:

- 2 avocados, pitted, and mashed
- ¼ teaspoon lemon stevia
- Salt and ground black pepper, to taste

- 1 tablespoon white vinegar
- 14 ounces coleslaw mix
- ¼ cup onion, chopped
- ¼ cup fresh cilantro, chopped
- Juice from 2 limes
- 2 tablespoons olive oil

Directions:
1. Put the coleslaw mixture in a salad bowl.
2. Add the avocado mash and onions, and toss to coat.
3. In a bowl, mix the lime juice with salt, pepper, oil, vinegar, and stevia, and stir well.
4. Add this to salad, toss to coat, sprinkle cilantro, and serve.

Nutrition:

Calories - 100, Fat - 10, Fiber - 2, Carbs - 5, Protein - 8

Creamy Celery Soup

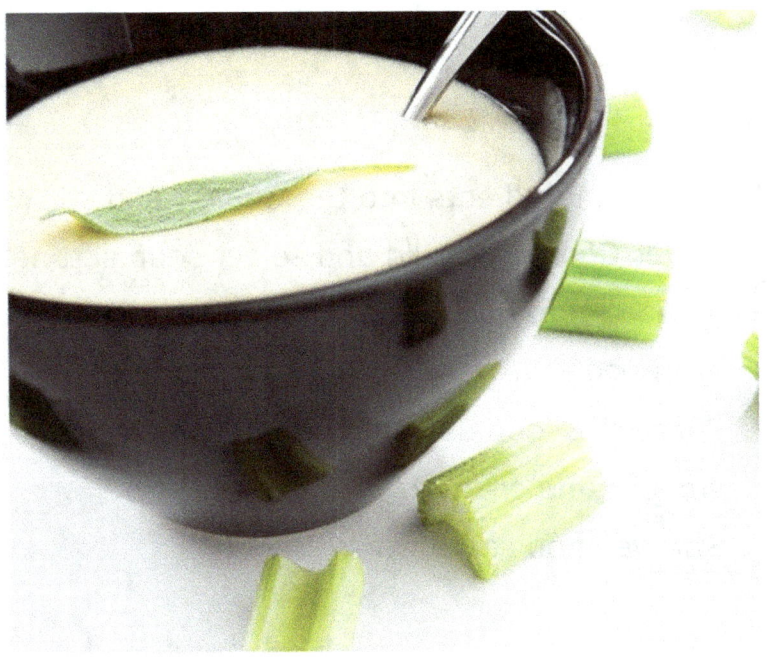

Preparation Time: 15 minutes

Cooking Time: 25 minutes

Servings: 4

Ingredients:

- 6 cups celery
- ½ tsp dill
- 1 onion, chopped

- 2 cups water
- 1 cup coconut milk
- Pinch of salt

Directions:

1. Add all ingredients into the Cooker and stir well.
2. Cover Cooker with lid and select soup setting.
3. Release pressure using quick release method than open the lid.
4. Puree the soup using an immersion blender until smooth and creamy.
5. Stir well and serve warm.

Nutrition:

Calories 174, Fat 14.6g, Carbohydrates 10.5g, Sugar 5.2g, Protein 2.8g, Cholesterol 0mg

Curried Butternut And Red Lentil Soup With Chard

Preparation time: 5 minutes

cooking time: 55 minutes

servings: 4

Ingredients

- 1 tablespoon olive oil
- 1 medium onion, chopped
- 1 tablespoon minced fresh ginger
- 1 tablespoon hot or mild curry powder
- 1 medium butternut squash, peeled and diced
- 1 garlic clove, minced
- 1 (14.5-ounce can crushed tomatoes
- 3 cups chopped stemmed Swiss chard
- 1 cup red lentils, picked over, rinsed, and drained
- 5 cups vegetable broth, homemade (see Light Vegetable Broth or store-bought, or water
- Salt and freshly ground black pepper

Directions

1. In a large soup pot, heat the oil over medium heat. Add the onion, squash, and garlic.
2. Cover and cook until softened, about 10 minutes.
3. Stir in the ginger and curry powder, then add the tomatoes, lentils, broth, and salt and pepper to taste.
4. Bring to boil, then reduce heat to low and simmer, uncovered, until the lentils and vegetables are tender, occasionally stirring, about 45 minutes.
5. About 15 minutes before serving, stir in the chard. Taste, adjusting seasonings if necessary, and serve.

Spinach, Walnut, And Apple Soup

Preparation time: 10 minutes

cooking time: 20 minutes

servings: 4

Ingredients

- 1 tablespoon olive oil
- 1 small onion, chopped
- 3 cups vegetable broth, homemade (see Light Vegetable Broth or store-bought, or water
- 2 Fuji or other flavorful apples
- 4 cups fresh spinach
- 1 teaspoon minced fresh sage or 1/2 teaspoon dried
- 1/4 teaspoon ground allspice
- 1 cup apple juice
- ¾ cup ground walnuts
- Salt and freshly ground black pepper
- 1 cup soy milk
- 1/4 cup toasted walnut pieces

Directions

1. In a large soup pot, heat the oil over medium heat. Add the onion, cover, and cook until softened, 5 minutes. Add about 1 cup of the vegetable broth, cover, and cook until the onion is very soft, about 5 minutes longer.
2. Peel, core, and chop one of the apples and add it to the pot with the onion and broth. Add the apple juice, spinach, ground walnuts, sage, allspice, the remaining 2 cups broth, and salt and pepper to taste. Bring to a boil, then reduce heat to low and simmer for 10 minutes.
3. Puree the soup in the pot with an immersion blender or in a blender or food processor, in batches if necessary, and return to the pot. Stir in the soy milk and reheat over medium heat until hot.
4. Chop the remaining apple. Ladle the soup into bowls, garnish each bowl with some of the chopped apple, sprinkle with the walnut pieces, and serve.

Tuscan White Bean Soup

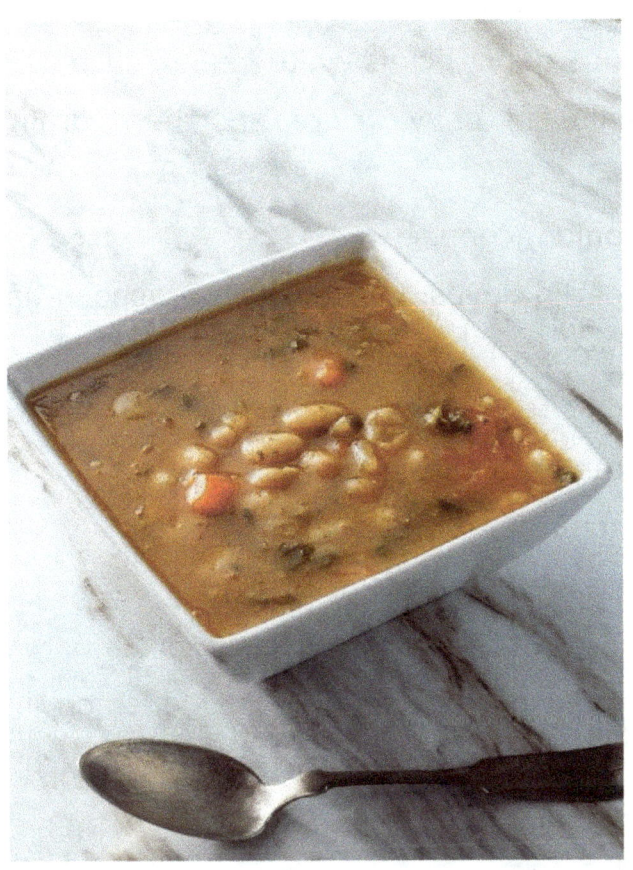

Preparation Time: 10 Minutes

Cooking Time: 15 Minutes

Servings:4

Ingredients

- 1 to 2 teaspoons olive oil
- 2 carrots, peeled and chopped
- 2 (15-ounce) cans white beans, such as cannellini, navy, or great northern, drained and rinsed
- 1 onion, chopped
- 4 garlic cloves, minced, or 1 teaspoon garlic powder
- Salt
- 1 tablespoon dried herbs
- Pinch freshly ground black pepper
- Pinch red pepper flakes
- 4 cups Economical Vegetable Broth or water
- 2 tablespoons freshly squeezed lemon juice
- 2 cups chopped greens, such as spinach, kale, arugula, or chard

Directions

1. Preparing the Ingredients.
2. Heat the olive oil in a large soup pot over medium-high heat.
3. Add the onion, garlic (if using fresh), carrots, and a pinch of salt.

4. Sauté for about 5 minutes, stirring occasionally, until the vegetables are lightly browned. Sprinkle in the dried herbs (plus the garlic powder, if using), black pepper, and red pepper flakes, and toss to combine.
5. Add the vegetable broth, beans, and another pinch of salt, and bring the soup to a low simmer to heat through. If you like, make the broth a bit creamier by puréeing 1 to 2 cups of soup in a countertop blender and returning it to the pot. Alternatively, use a hand blender to purée about one-fourth of the beans in the pot.
6. Stir in the lemon juice and greens, and let the greens wilt into the soup before serving.
7. Leftovers can be kept in an airtight container for up to 1 week in the refrigerator or up to 1 month in the freezer.

Nutrition Per Serving (2 cups)

Calories: 145; Protein: 7g; Total fat: 2g; Saturated fat: 0g; Carbohydrates: 26g; Fiber: 6g

Cream of Tomato Soup

Preparation Time: 5 Minutes

Cooking Time: 5 Minutes

Servings: 2

Ingredients

- 1 (28-ounce) can crushed, diced, or whole peeled tomatoes, undrained
- ¾ to 1 cup unsweetened nondairy milk
- 1 to 2 teaspoons dried herbs
- 2 to 3 teaspoons onion powder (optional)
- ½ teaspoon salt, or to taste
- Freshly ground black pepper

Directions

1. Preparing the Ingredients.
2. Pour the tomatoes and their juices into a large pot and bring them to near-boiling over medium heat.
3. Add the dried herbs, onion powder (if using), milk, salt, and pepper to taste.
4. Stir to combine.

5. If you used diced or whole tomatoes, use a hand blender to purée the soup until smooth. (Alternatively, let the soup cool for a few minutes, then transfer to a countertop blender.)
6. Leftovers will keep in an airtight container for up to 1 week in the refrigerator or up to 1 month in the freezer (though if you want leftovers for this soup, you might want to double the recipe).

Nutrition Per Serving (2 cups)

Calories: 90; Protein: 4g; Total fat: 3g; Saturated fat: 0g; Carbohydrates: 16g; Fiber: 4g

Chickpea, Tomato, And Eggplant Stew

Preparation Time: 5 Minutes

Cooking Time: 55 Minutes

Servings: 4

Ingredients

- 1 tablespoon olive oil
- 1 large onion, chopped
- 1 medium eggplant, peeled and cut into 1/2-inch dice
- 2 medium carrots, cut into 1/4-inch slices
- 1 medium red bell pepper, cut into 1-inch dice
- 1 large Yukon Gold potato, peeled and cut into 1/2-inch dice
- 3 garlic cloves, minced
- 2 cups cooked or 1 (15.5-ounce) cans chickpeas, drained and rinsed if canned
- 1 (28-ounce) can diced tomatoes, undrained
- 1 tablespoon minced fresh parsley
- 1/2 teaspoon dried oregano
- 1/2 teaspoon dried basil
- 1 tablespoon soy sauce

www.ingramcontent.com/pod-product-compliance
Lightning Source LLC
Chambersburg PA
CBHW070102120526
44589CB00033B/1479